Small Guide for the Camino de Santiago
Written and illustrated by Julie Maggi
Copyright © Julie Maggi 2024
All rights reserved



This book was painted entirely by hand.



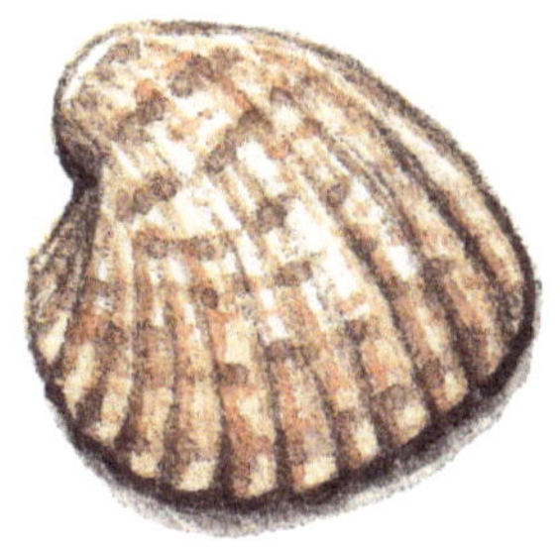

More than ten years ago, when I created the first version of this little guide, I didn't have the hiking experience that I have now, just a lot of enthusiasm and curiosity.

Since then, I have walked the French Way, the English Way, the Via de la Plata and the Sanabrese Way (all in Spain), the Via Francigena in Italy, the Thames Path in England, the Rheinsteig in Germany and many other smaller routes around Europe (The travel diaries relating to my journeys to Santiago are available on Amazon).

The style of my illustrations has matured a lot over the years and I understood that I could offer a book written and painted with more attention to detail. I used my own handmade watercolours (which are available for purchase on my website www.juliemaggi.com) and watercolour pencils (Albrecht Dürer by Faber-Castell).

I hope you will enjoy it.

Julie Maggi

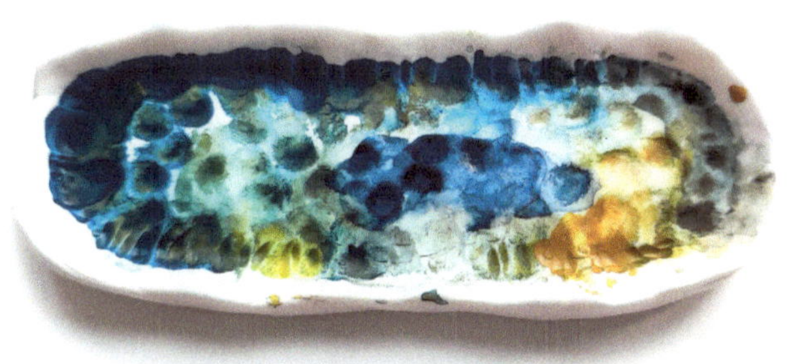

I hope that one day you too can travel these paths and find answers to questions you didn't know you had.

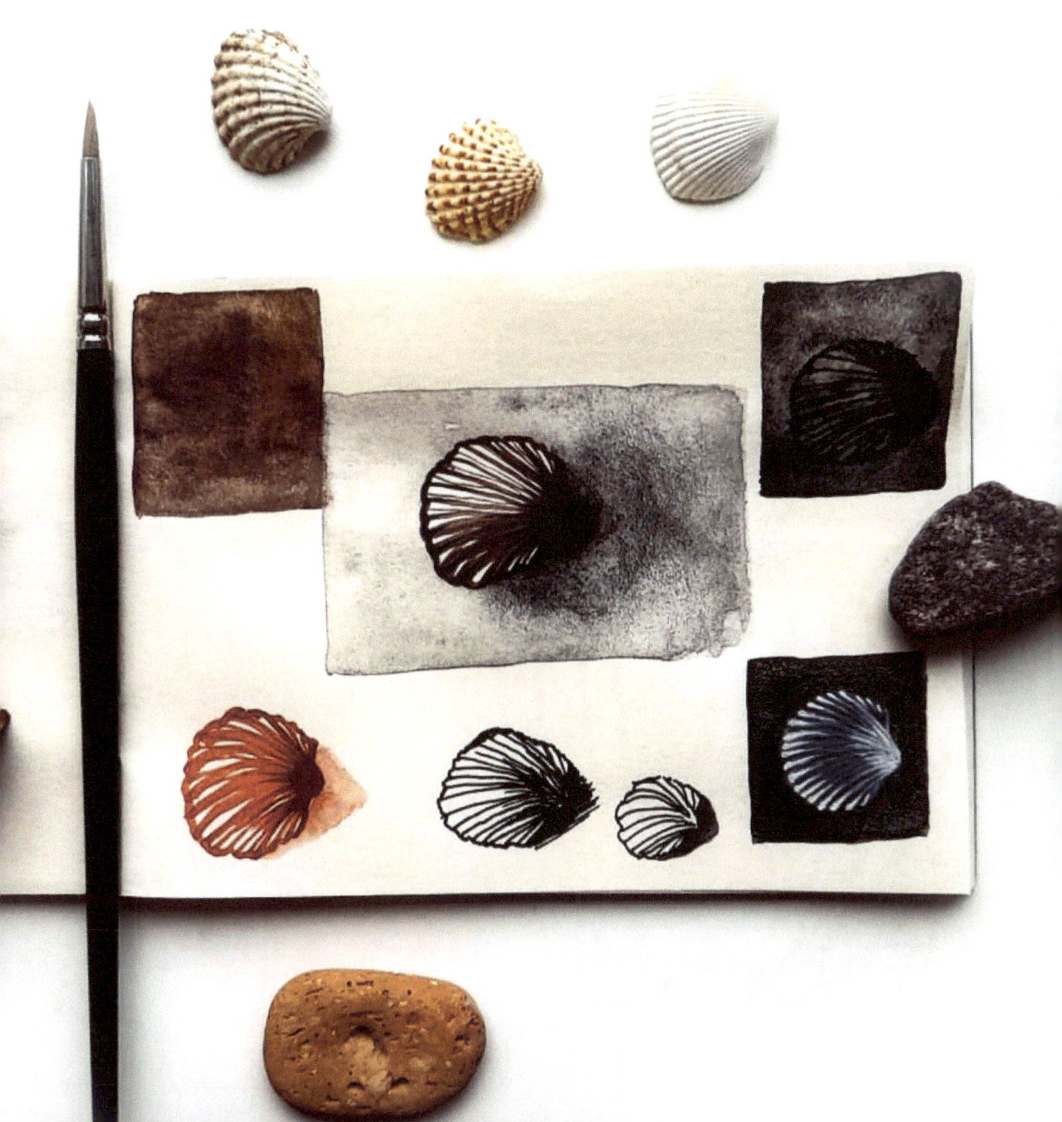

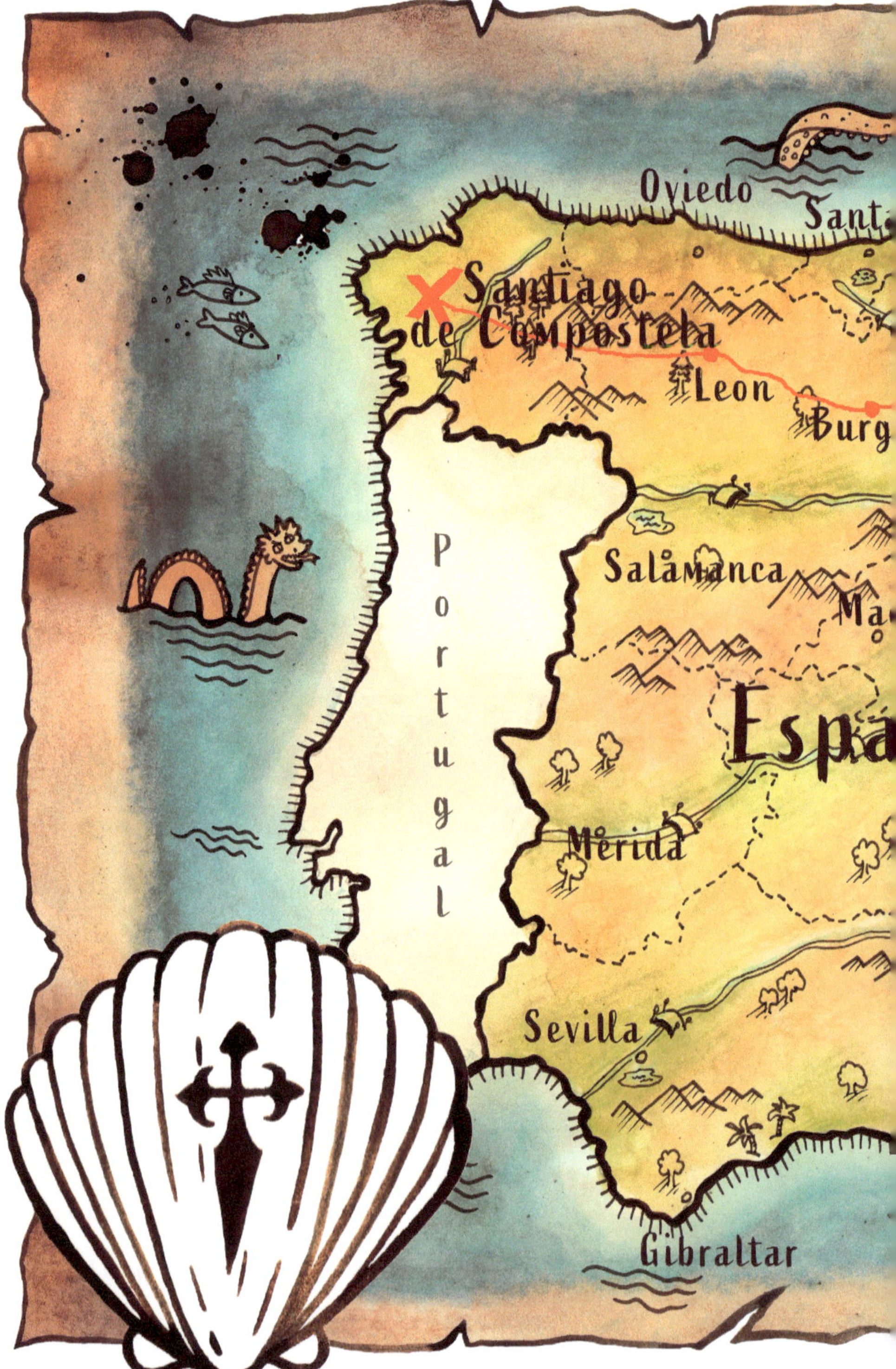

Oviedo
Sant
Santiago
de Compostela
Leon
Burg
Portugal
Salamanca
Ma
Espa
Mérida
Sevilla
Gibraltar

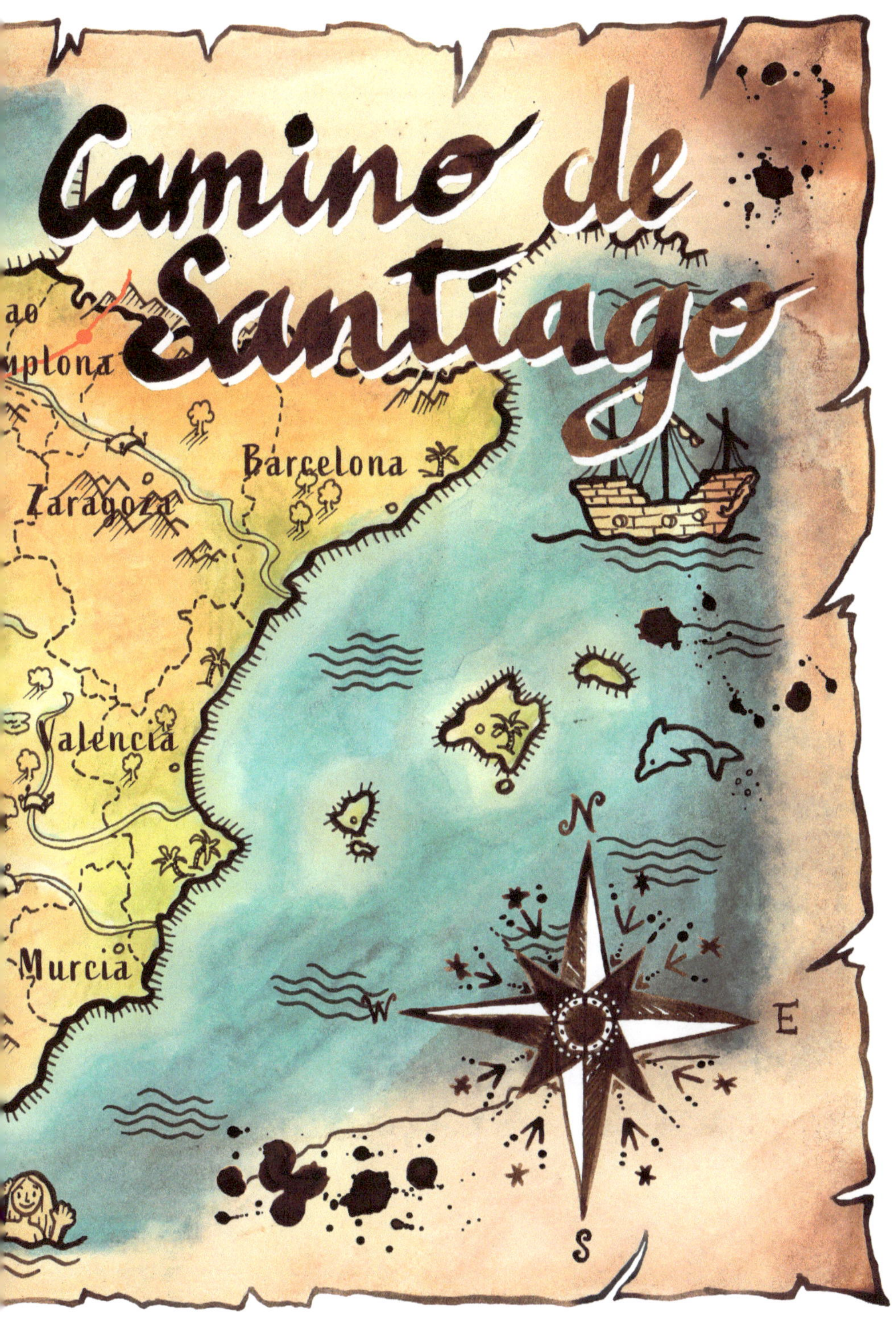

Camino de Santiago
ao
mplona
Barcelona
Zaragoza
Valencia
Murcia
N
W
E
S

The legend of Santiago's life is full of interesting details and full of historical references. It is said that the apostle James the Great, after travelling through Spain to Galicia to share the teachings of Christ, returned to his native Palestine. It was in his homeland that he was beheaded by King Herod Agrippa in the year 44, thus becoming the first martyr apostle of Christianity. His disciples managed to steal his body and transported it, by boat, to Galicia where they buried him.

Centuries passed and every trace of the burial site was lost. Then, one night in the year 813, Pelagius the Hermit noticed lights similar to stars illuminating a field on Mount Liberon. In this place the remains of the Saint were found enclosed in a Roman-era tomb and also containing two other bodies as well as an inscription which indicated the name of the apostle.

The place was called campus stellae (from which the name "Santiago de Compostela" or "St. James of the field of stars" derives). It was precisely there that the cathedral of Santiago was built in 1075 to preserve the relics of the Saint. The cult of the apostle spread rapidly, becoming an integral part of Galicia's regional identity.

In 1987, the Council of Europe recognized the importance of the religious and cultural routes that cross Europe to reach Santiago de Compostela and declared the Way of Santiago "Cultural Route". In 1993, the roads travelled by pilgrims in France and Spain were declared a World Heritage Site by UNESCO. Thanks to the European commitment, many people have had the opportunity to walk the Camino for a variety of reasons both religious and cultural.

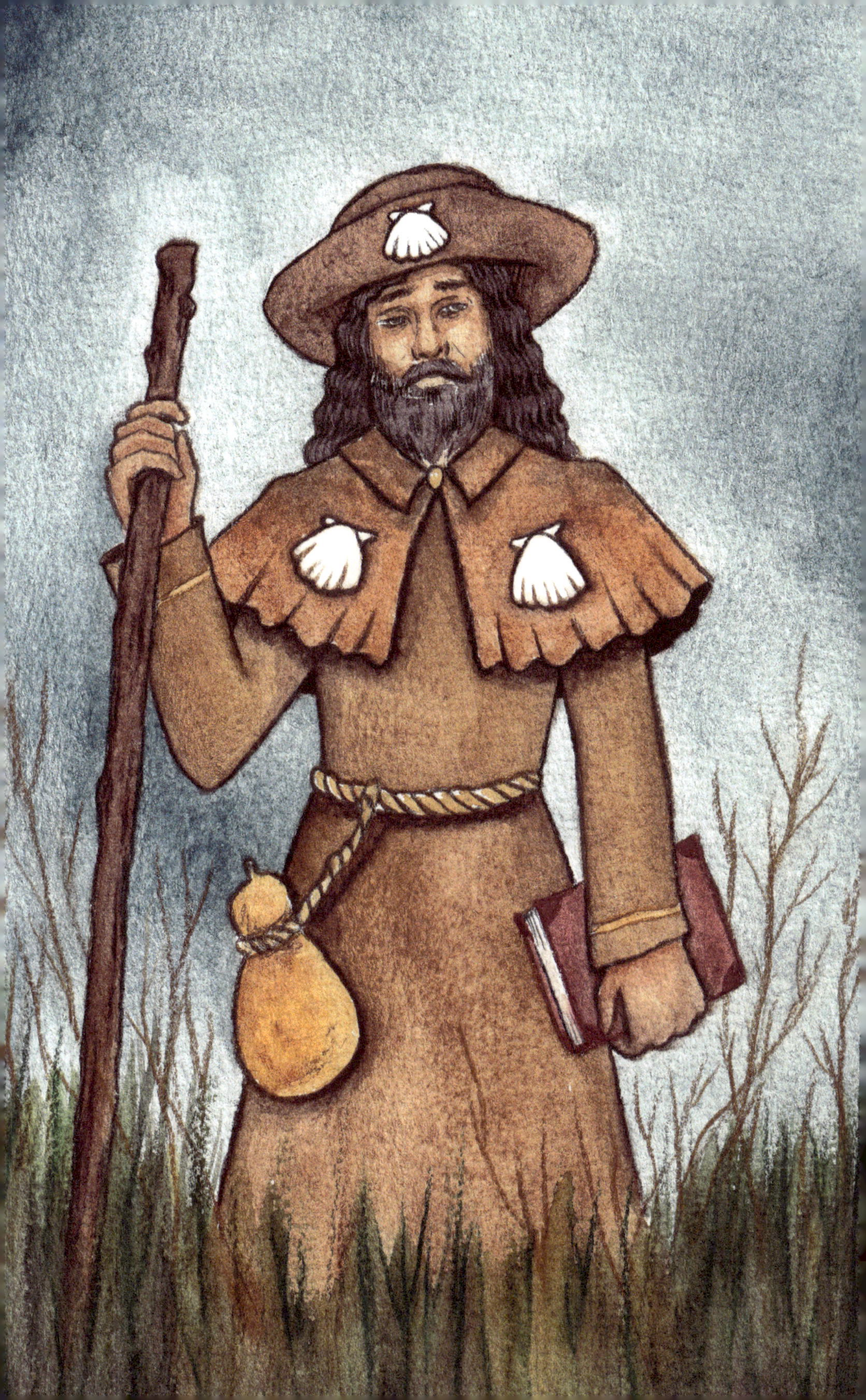

1. Focus on the movements and feel the muscles

In everyday life, we are constantly distracted and, unless we are in a gym or attend a yoga class, we do not give much thought to the movements of our body. When we walk the Camino everything changes: after a few kilometres, we will notice a certain tiredness in the muscles that we usually use less frequently. For some people it is a real discovery and we sometimes hear people saying "I didn't know I had a muscle there." Only a person who has a past as an athlete will be able to automatically connect the mind and the body. For all those who use their muscles to move around in everyday tasks, without pushing themselves beyond their limits, the Camino de Santiago will offer a great challenge: being able to maintain the balance between the need to cover numerous kilometres with a backpack on one's shoulder and the need to rest when necessary.

In the many journeys I have completed, I have had various difficulties with my muscles. Especially during the first few days, the idea of stopping to rest and losing a day of walking seemed absurd to me. I wanted to be strong and fast, without realizing that I was asking too much of my body. Only after several days of constant walking, the legs begin to strengthen: but the muscles need rest to regenerate!

My advice is to start the walk with short distances and increase the number of kilometres day by day. During the first day of my very first walk along the French Way, I only covered eight kilometres: I felt like a novice, but I couldn't do differently. Around me there were people of all ages and physical fitness: from young people in their twenties, fast and lively, to elderly retired walkers, sometimes more trained and sometimes less. I wasn't the only one who decided to stop after a short walk. Often, along the various routes, I came across pilgrims who didn't want to stop and rest: out of pride or haste they didn't understand that they were endangering the entire success of their undertaking. It happened to me more than once that I found them stuck in the subsequent stages, with major muscular problems. To avoid this type of inconvenience it is necessary to give maximum priority to listening to your body. A small pain may just be a symptom of tiredness, but it could, if not treated, turn into an obstacle that will make you return home sooner than expected.

2. Learn to take blisters seriously

As much as I love walking long distances, I have always suffered (and always will suffer) from blisters on my feet. It doesn't make any difference if the shoes are worn-in or brand new, breathable or padded: not even using the terrible trekking sandals with socks allowed me to walk the Camino from start to end without suffering from some blisters. Many people, usually people who have never travelled more than four kilometres in a row, told me: "It's not a big deal! It's just a blister on the foot!" Clearly, their ignorance regarding walking does not allow them to fully understand the gravity of the problem. Not only can a blister on the foot, if left untreated, turn into a nasty infection, but it can also lead to tendonitis. When we walk with a blister on our foot, we will involuntarily try to avoid putting our weight on the irritated area. This will cause an unnatural position of the foot which, in the long run, especially over several kilometres and many days of walking, will lead to inevitable inflammation of the tendons and at that point there is a big risk.

During a ten-kilometre running race in Vienna, I began to feel some pain in the anterior tibial tendon, in the front part of the leg that goes from the knee to the foot. I ignored the signs and continued running: I had trained for months and did not want to give in to something that could only be a temporary pain. I arrived at the end of the race in such pain that I immediately had to take a painkiller and for the next three months didn't touch my running shoes. If something like this happens on the walk, we might as well book a flight home. If there is a blister, or pain of any kind, it is important to treat the area immediately, with plasters and disinfectants or with ice packs and rest. There is no shortage of medical practices along the way and it is possible to benefit from hospital medical assistance if necessary. I have been to hospitals several times during my journey and not only will the doctors help you heal, but they will give you valuable advice so that you can continue along the path with fewer problems.

3. Use poles (they take off 20/30% of the weight of the backpack)

During my first walk I decided to carry a thirteen-kilo backpack on my shoulders. I had no idea that this was too heavy and after a few days of walking, I started to feel pain everywhere along my spine. An older pilgrim advised me to find some trekking poles. This was a rather difficult undertaking in the middle of nowhere, surrounded by the countryside of La Rioja, which is not exactly famous for its forest areas. My travel companion at the time found a stick along the road and, after cleaning it, used it along the way: it was certainly heavier than a set of technical poles, but it did its job. I decided to do the same. It is no coincidence that we see images of pilgrims always accompanied by a walking stick: it is truly an indispensable aid, especially for those, like me, who suffer from back problems. During one of the first stages of my walk along the Plata, I received a technical trekking pole as a gift. The hospitalero who gave me the stick knew the route I was about to follow very well (dirt road with a steep slope) and, seeing me without support, had decided to give me one of the many technical sticks that pilgrims forget in the albergues or along the Path. Since then, I have never stopped using it: it has improved my balance, helped me avoid multiple injuries and improved my posture. Of course, now my backpack weighs a maximum of four and a half kilos, but I never leave my trekking pole behind and my body is grateful for that.

4. Leave early in the morning to avoid suffering from the heat

Spain, like the entire Mediterranean, becomes scorching hot in summer: whether it is the North or the South, temperatures go above 40°C. Walking under the sun with such high temperatures means risking sunstroke, sunburn and makes it mandatory to carry several litres of water, which increases the weight of the backpack. I learned the hard way that arriving at the hostel before lunchtime offers a whole series of benefits. If we travel four kilometres per hour and have to cover a distance of twenty-five kilometres, then this translates into six and a half hours (or rather seven, to add a break) of walking. Thus, if we are leaving at five in the morning we will arrive at noon. Early risers will have no problem waking up when it's still dark outside and setting off before the sun has begun its journey across the sky. For those who like to wake up calmly, this could be a good time to challenge themselves. Jokes aside: the reasons why I strongly recommend setting off very early are various and don't just have to do with temperatures.

Arriving at the hostel before midday, you have time to stop by a few shops and buy some food. In Spain, from two to five in the afternoon, businesses take a break to enjoy a siesta. If you arrive late, you will find everything closed and end up having to wait a long time before being able to do your shopping. Another valid reason is that, especially in recent years, the number of pilgrims has increased exponentially. By taking it easy, you risk arriving at the hostel and not finding a place to sleep.

The last valid reason for arriving at the hostel when the sun is still high in the sky is the need to wash your clothes and let them dry in the sun. Many hostels don't have a dryer and, even when they do, it often doesn't work very well. I'm not a big fan of dryers: they ruin fabrics and usually don't leave a good smell on clothes, especially when they are used by hundreds of pilgrims a week, without receiving the necessary maintenance. By arriving at the hostel early, you can use the time available to wash your clothes and let them dry in the sun or wring them out with a towel and hang them on your bed.

5. Buy excellent quality shoes and use them before starting the Camino

My first piece of advice regarding the shoes for the Camino is to take them a size and a half larger. During the long hours of walking up and down the hills, sometimes under the scorching sun, the feet swell from fatigue and the heat. Wearing a pair of "large" shoes allows the foot to have space to grow during the journey: it seems hard to believe but from the first to the last day of walking, the foot grows. Why is that? It's actually quite simple: feet include bones, tendons and muscles, so day after day, movement after movement, the muscles of the feet develop, the tendons strengthen and lengthen and so, even if not very noticeable, our feet grow by several millimetres.

Wearing shoes that are loose also allows you to have space to use the double sock technique. During my first walk, I met a Swiss soldier who suggested this technique to me, useful for mitigating the damage caused by blisters. You should wear a lighter, softer sock in contact with the skin and a sturdier, more padded sock in contact with the shoe. I must say that, although it is annoying to have to get used to this routine, after a few days you notice the difference. Another piece of advice regarding the type of shoe to buy is to choose the Gore-Tex version only and exclusively if you plan to travel in a very rainy season. During the summer, it rains very little in Spain and waterproof shoes will overheat your feet unnecessarily. Along the Plata, I tried the minimalist shoes with the Vibram sole and must say that those felt very good. The only downside is that it is easier for pebbles or wild grass to slip in, but it doesn't take much to get rid of them. It is clear that depending on the terrain, the type of footwear needed also changes. Along the first stages of the French Way, one crosses the Pyrenees, thus climbing mountains, with the possibility of getting

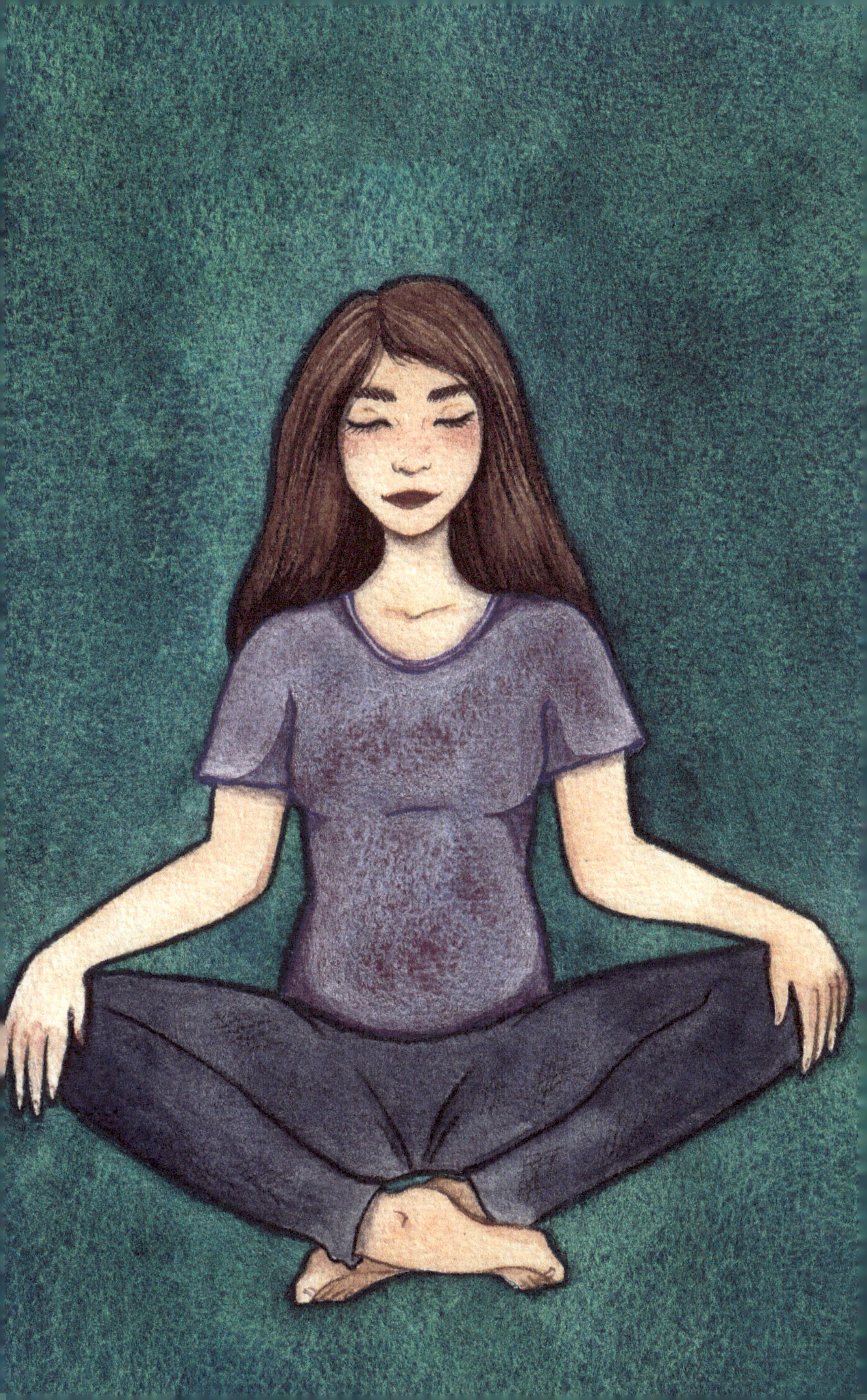

sprained or encountering vipers (I have met several along my various routes, in Spain and in other parts of Europe). Therefore, it is advisable to use mountain boots, which support the ankle and better protect against possible sprains. Once you have completed the steeper stages, you can send a package to your home address, containing what you no longer need, including shoes. I did just that, along the Plata, getting rid of a kilo and a half of objects that I wasn't using anymore.

6. After each stage do stretching exercises

For many years, I have been practicing yoga and pilates regularly, several times a week and learned to stretch my muscles to help my body stay healthy. Stretching helps to increase flexibility which is absolutely necessary to avoid injuries, especially when travelling on unpaved roads, steep descents or slippery paths. Being able to move the joints of our body without problems allows us to make movements that would otherwise be difficult: lift the backpack from the ground, take a jump to avoid a hole, pull ourselves up without needing help. Muscles and tendons stiffen with age. It is necessary not only to do a whole series of exercises to help protect the elasticity of the tissues, but also to facilitate the dispersion of lactic acid.
Furthermore, the stretching of the muscles that occurs after a targeted exercise also leads to greater relaxation during rest, which is the perfect way to allow the body to regenerate. I have discovered that the first four kilometres of walking are always the most difficult: the body seems asleep and tense.

For me, everything improved with the following routine: I start walking without haste, for about twenty minutes. At that point, I stop, put down my backpack and do some stretching. I immediately notice that my legs get rid of that feeling of heaviness and stiffness, and my back benefits too. Then, at the end of the daily stage, I repeat the procedure, adding a nice massage to the sore spots. I usually use alcohol de romero (rosemary alcohol), a panacea for feet and legs that can be purchased at the pharmacy.

7. Don't tie yourself to anyone who doesn't have your walking speed

Imagine meeting a very nice person along the way with whom you get along quickly and who makes you laugh and pass the time. Between one chat and another the kilometres fly by and in no time, you have arrived at your destination. You start walking together but, after a few days, you realize that this person is much better trained than you and is slowing down his pace to be able to walk alongside you. This is what happened to me during the first stages of my first Camino. The person in question was a twenty-three-year-old man (I was twenty-nine) who is still my best friend. When I realized that I was slowing him down, I decided to change the way we managed our walking days. We agreed to always stop together, but to walk separately: it was the best choice we could have made and it saved us a lot of frustration. Unless it was decided at the start to walk the Camino with a person who for one reason or another is slower or has different habits than us (for example, someone who needs to stop often for a cigarette or for a coffee break in a bar) it is really difficult to find a compromise. Along other paths, I happened to make friends with people who loved to sleep late: the first few days I tried to wait for them, but then I realized that this type of organization wasn't good for me, as I suffer a lot from the heat at noon. Agree to meet at the end of the stage so you can share a meal (and maybe even a room in the hostel to share the place with someone who isn't a complete stranger) and the freedom to walk at your own pace is, at least in my opinion, the best solution.

8. Take long walks before setting off on the Camino

When I realized I wanted to walk my first Camino; I was in Turin. I was a student at the Academy of Fine Arts and, spending most of my days sitting in class or sitting at my desk studying and preparing for exams, I didn't have a very trained body. Before embarking on the undertaking of crossing Spain on foot, I chose to train for the challenge. I signed up for a bike-sharing program and started (with a lot of effort) running. Whenever possible, I tried to use my free time during the weekends, to go on long walks. First, right along the river, then up to the neighbouring town. I tried to join groups of people who were enthusiastic about the mountains. Thus, I arrived at my first day of walking with at least a minimum of preparation. A fundamental thing to do is to wear the same shoes that you intend to use along the Camino route. If they are uncomfortable, you always have time to buy new ones and, if not, you will already have them broken in ready when the real journey begins.

9. Have your feet checked by an expert (beautician or podiatrist)

Blisters aside, I've never had any major difficulties related to my feet: no particular orthopaedic complications and, until now, no mycosis or skin inflammation due to bacteria. But I must say that I am very careful about foot care: I use comfortable shoes, almost always open, I never use heels and I do pedicures regularly. In any case, before starting even just training, I recommend having your feet checked: if an orthopaedic insole or specific treatment for some toenails with suspicious stains is necessary, it is better to do so ahead of the walk. Often, when we lack experience, we cut our toenails incorrectly and sometimes we encourage abnormal growths and infections. For this reason, asking a beautician to take care of your pedicure for the weeks before the walk can help you avoid obstacles along the way. Of all the impediments that can arise during the Camino, those related to the feet are the most frequent, but they can often be averted by asking an expert for assistance. Setting a specific budget for foot-care, even while walking, is the best way to avoid annoying pain and complications (you will find beauty centres specialized in foot care in the larger cities along the entire route).

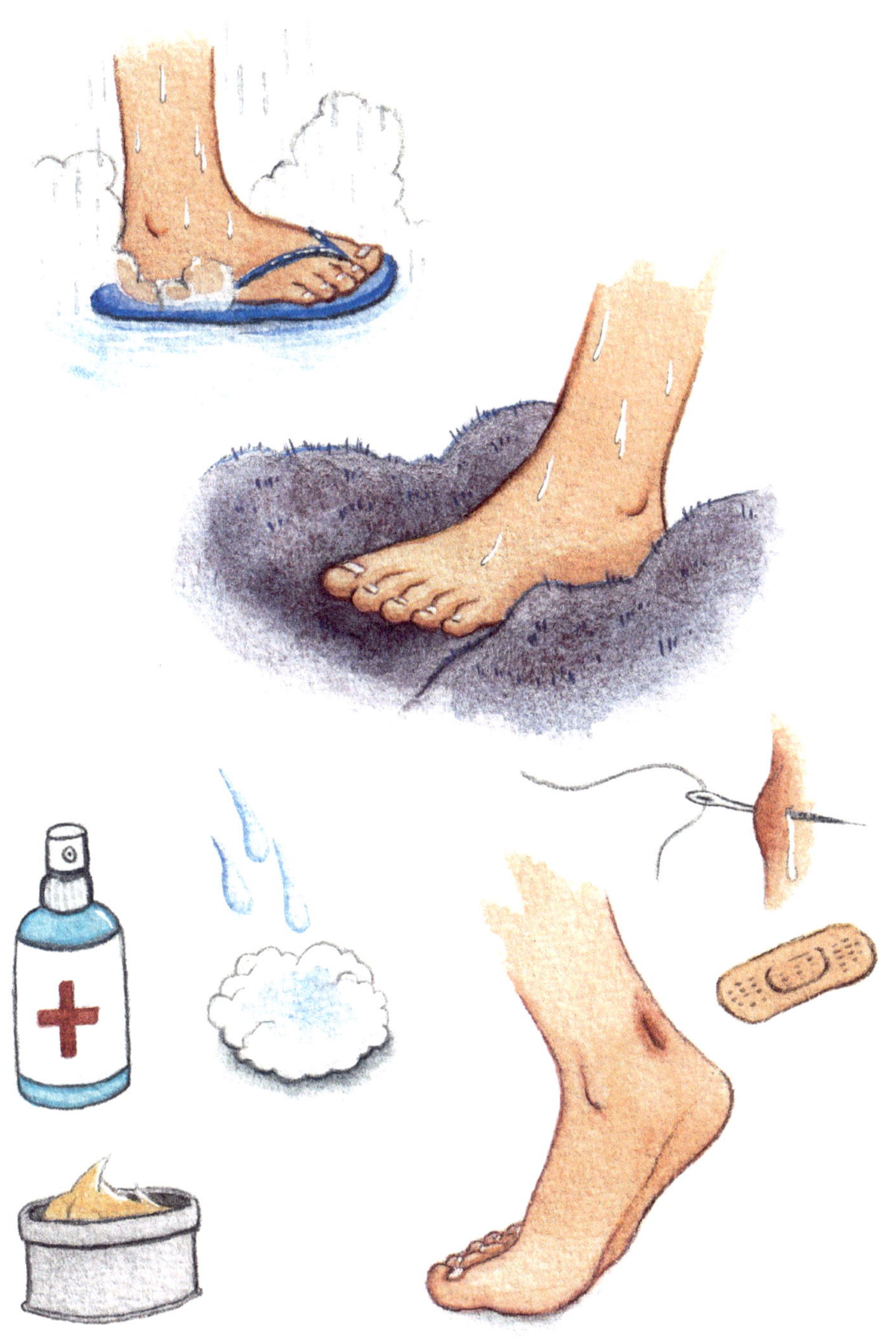

10. If possible, in the months before departure, forget about cars and buses

When it is not possible to use the weekends to train by going to the mountains with a backpack on your shoulders, the best thing to do is to just walk as much as possible. Going to the supermarket or to work: every step counts. Try downloading an application that counts your steps – you will be amazed to check your statistics. On average, during a day away from home it is easy to exceed ten thousand steps (which is an excellent amount if you want to maintain leg health and good blood circulation).

There are also machines that allow you to simulate the movement of walking in the mountains. If you don't have the space to keep them at home you might consider joining a gym. Not only treadmills, but also elliptical machines are very helpful to prepare you for the walk. Furthermore, do squats and lunges, to keep your muscles active even without walking, especially if you have a sedentary job (I know something about this). It is important to find twenty minutes a day to move your legs.

If possible, use the backpack you plan to take with you on your journey to carry groceries or any other shopping. Use the same backpack also to go to work, to the swimming pool or to carry your belongings during a weekend trip. Your backpack will be your home (like a snail) during the weeks on the road. Learning the weaknesses and strengths of the backpack will help you find solutions before it's too late. For example, you might figure out that one of the shoulder straps scratches your left shoulder or that the bottom is not completely waterproof or that one of the zips is slightly defective. And maybe you'll decide to invest in a new backpack, like I did recently, after using the same one for more than ten years.

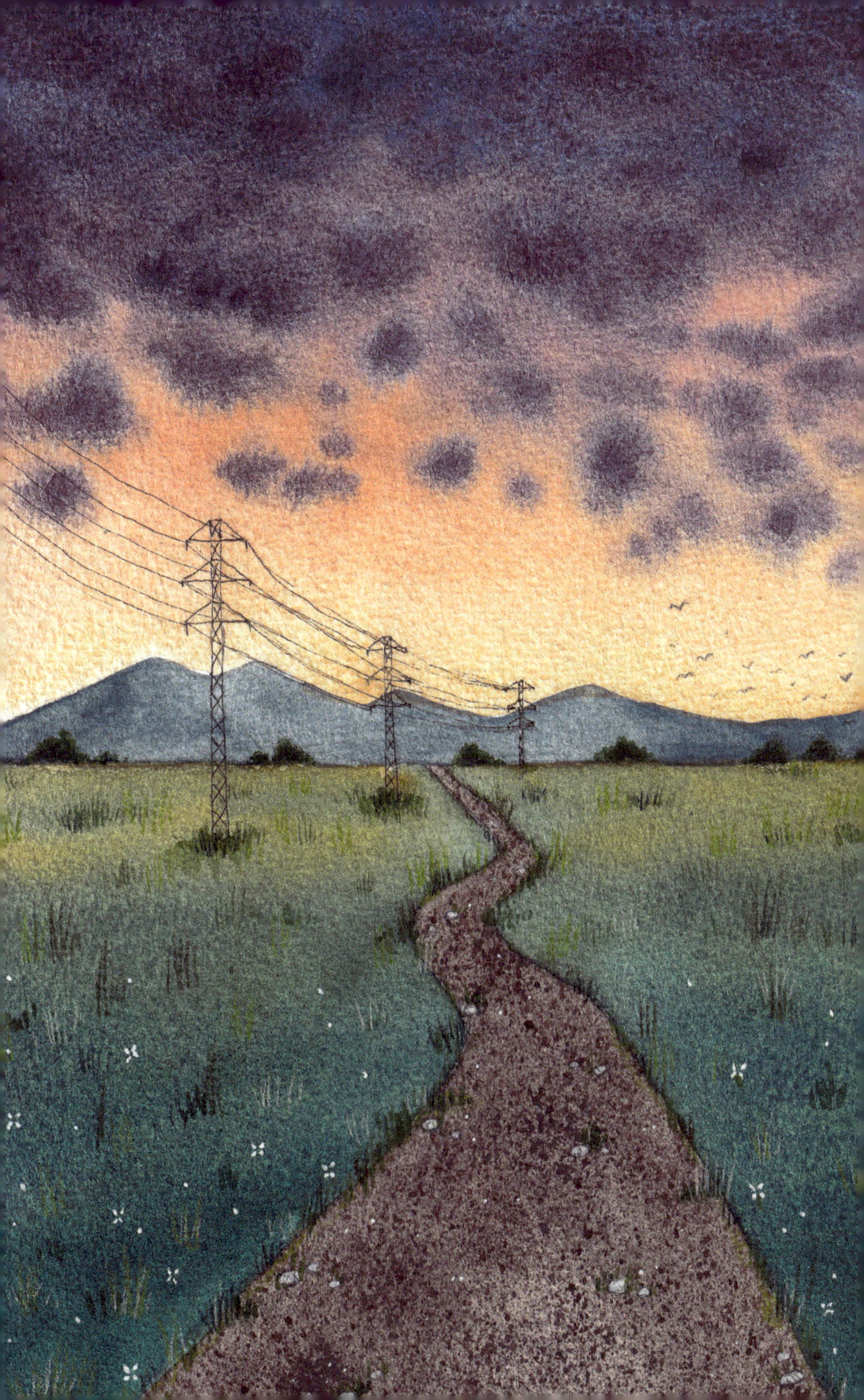

The experience of the Camino de Santiago is for many people a time of profound internal change. Keeping a diary allows you to retrace the stages of your journey and your personal evolution, once the journey is over, and to return, in your mind, to the most important places and moments. However, writing during the days of intense physical effort is not easy. At the end of the day, you often find yourself tired and unmotivated and you just want to take a shower, eat something and take a nap.
Keeping a daily diary is not impossible, you just need to follow a few simple tricks.

1. Bring a small notebook. This way it will be easier to transport and the thought of writing a page a day won't scare you. No one judges the quantity or quality of journal writing – it's a private place.

2. After having prioritized the most important actions such as eating or washing clothes at the end of the daily interval, once you are calm, decide to dedicate even just five minutes to writing. There is no need to list every single detail of the day: just the things that struck you most, that made you smile or moved you. The jokes of some other pilgrim or the food you ate, a particular place or the title of a song that got stuck in your head.

3. Always remember to add the date and location to each diary page.

4. For those who don't know how to start, it may be a good idea to pretend that the diary is an old friend. The diary could begin like this:

" Dear … I'm writing to tell you about my journey…"

5. Leave space to add small printed photos, such as polaroids.

Nowadays there are various applications that allow you to add cute graphics to photos taken with your mobile phone (for those who don't want to bring their camera along). Photos can later be printed and glued to the journal to add a personal touch to the pages.

I must warn lovers of en plein air painting that, with the limited time available during the Camino, it is not always possible to sit down and paint. An easier way to jot down some ideas on paper is to choose a faster and more immediate style, like the one used by urban sketching enthusiasts: you can select just one colour (personally, I really like sepia and diluted black watercolours and ink).
Technical drawing pencils and pens are also fine. In this sketch, I represented a detail of the baptismal font in the Bayonne Cathedral.

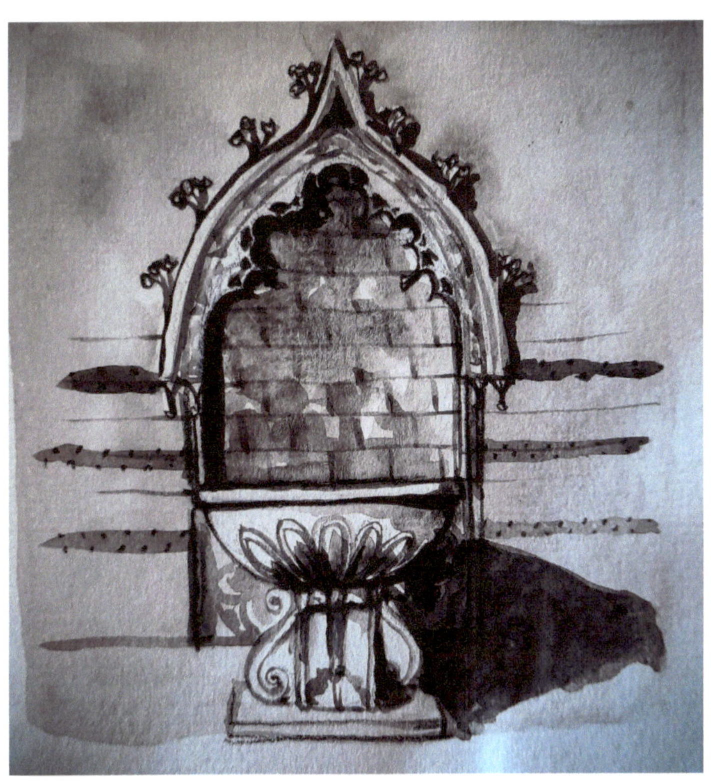

Painting can be a way to retrace in your mind the roads travelled along the Camino, once you return home. In images, I'll show you step by step how I created this simple illustration. First, we need to find a photo from our trip that inspires us. For me, a small stretch of road hugged by trees is very significant, because it reminds me of the relief I felt under that shade, after walking for hours and hours under the sun.

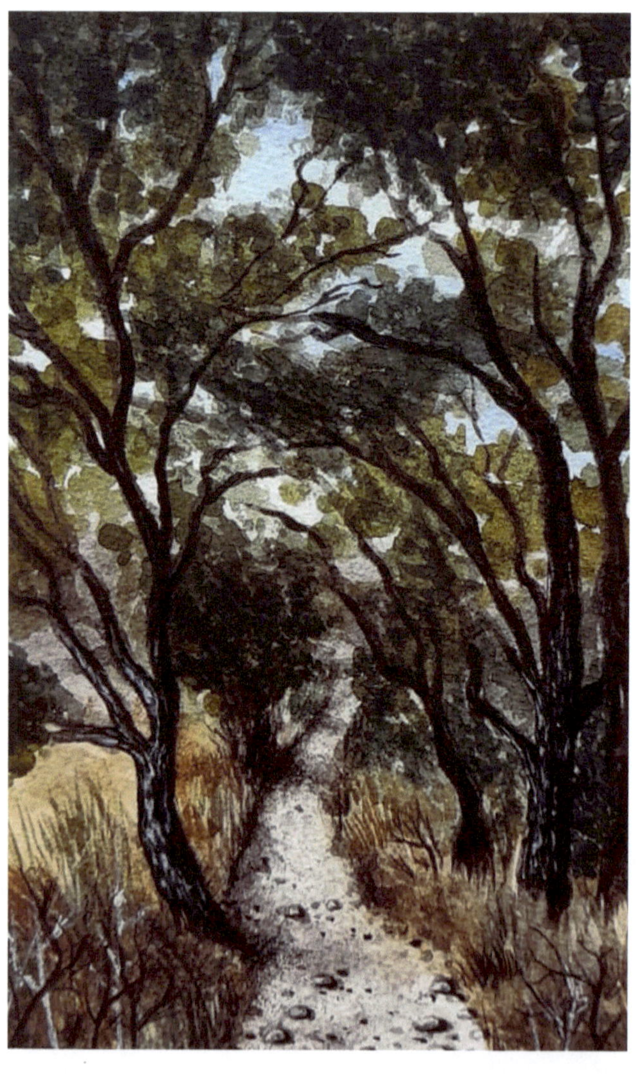

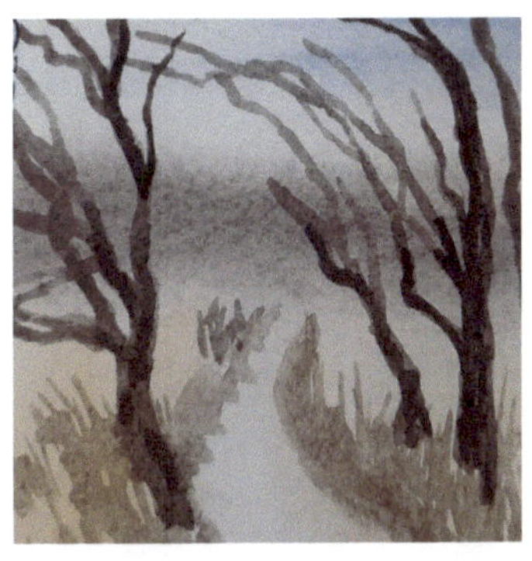

I used a very small palette, just shades of brown, ochre, green and a little blue. I didn't make a sketch but started from the essential shapes of the branches.

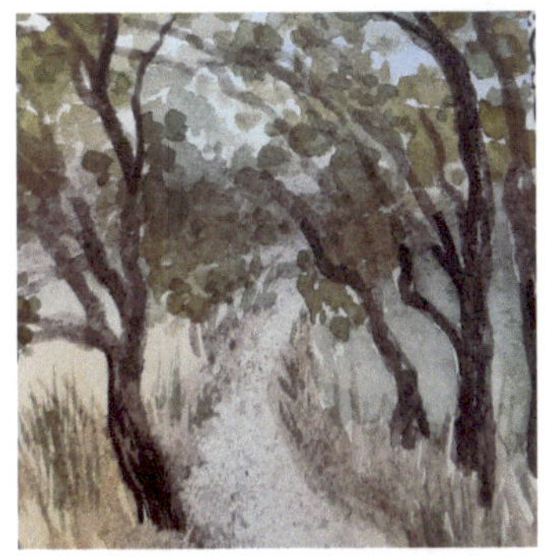

I added volumes, filling the spaces where the leaves grew with greater density.

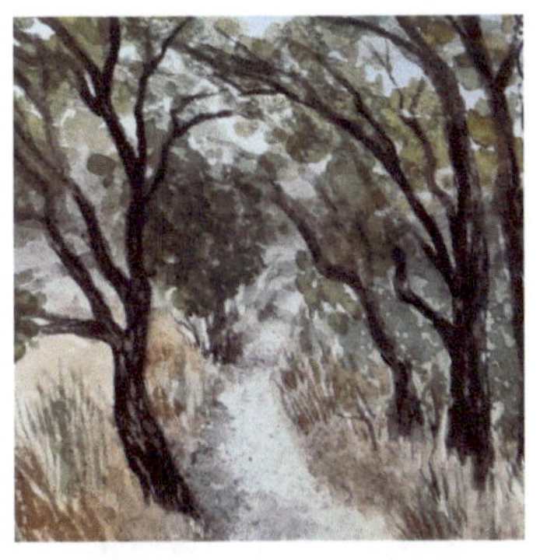

I then painted the tufts of dry grass that covered the ground, trying to give the idea of what was a country road.

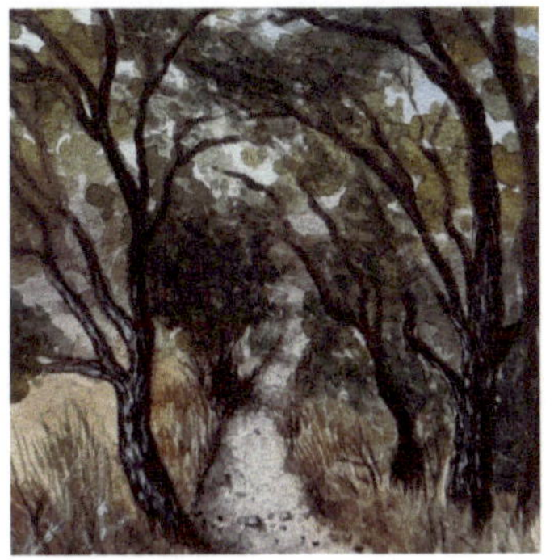

Finally, I outlined the shadows and details of the dirt road: I sprayed the colour with an old toothbrush and created darker areas with the help of a natural sponge.

Over the course of the several years that have passed between my first Camino and today, I found myself walking in completely different types of terrains, climates and altitudes, depending on the places I was in.

Along the French Way, the most frequented by pilgrims of all ages, the climate changes a lot depending on the region you are crossing. At the beginning of the route, while crossing the border between France and Spain, you find yourself walking in the mountains. There are those who have walked this path in winter and had to carry a backpack full of warm clothes and wool socks. Clearly, when travelled in winter, the path becomes lonely and it is easier to find a place to sleep in hostels (even if some close for the winter, so make sure to inform yourself in advance), but it becomes more difficult from a climate and clothing point of view as your clothes, for example, will take a long time to dry. I walked along the first stretch in mid-August and can say that, apart from a heavy sweatshirt and a pair of leggings, I didn't need any additional clothing.

I have learned that I prefer a good light poncho to a waterproof jacket, because it also covers the backpack and allows better breathability. If you are trying to save, both in terms of money and weight, I recommend disposable ponchos (which, if you are careful, can be folded up and actually be used numerous times). There are ponchos that also become "tarps", large waterproof sheets with a hole for the head, a hood and clips on the sides to close them around the body: they are useful and multifunctional (also for lying on the ground and taking a break), they can also be used if you decide to travel a short distance by bicycle, and even as an emergency shelter in case of sudden rain along the road. I appreciated the fact that I had a fleece-lined windbreaker with me, which also proved to be perfect for those temporary drizzles that can happen, especially in the Galicia area or on the Northern Way.

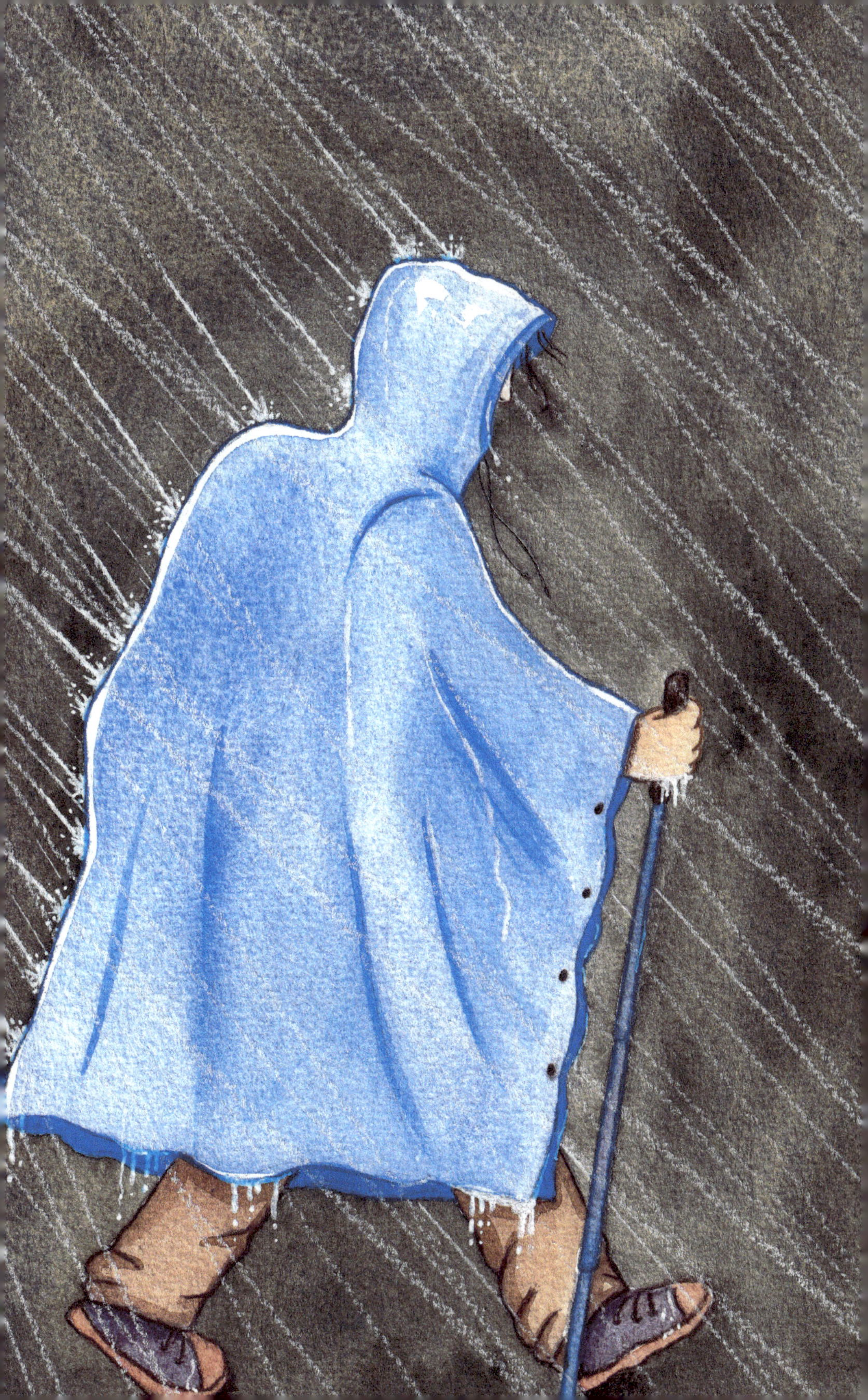

Along the French Way, you find yourself walking along the famous Mesetas, a very long expanse of wheat fields that continues for days and days of walking. During this part of the journey, you must be very careful not to get sunburnt, so carry enough water to drink, wear a hat with a visor and sunglasses, and, finally, always apply total sun protection. In some stages along the Plata, I feared I would die, due to the total lack of drinking water along routes of tens of kilometres: if travelled under the midday sun in August, ten kilometres could become fatal. I know that sounds like an exaggeration but it's not. Just look at the sides of the road and you can often see the tombstones of pilgrims who didn't make it.

Waking up early in the morning, you will travel the first kilometres in the dark, often on roads made of dirt. Since you frequently come across tractors and other agricultural vehicles at that time, it can happen that they raise a lot of dust and make breathing more difficult. A system that works wonderfully is that of carrying a sterile mask with you (I think we all know where to find them nowadays) to take out when necessary. It is also useful to wear it if you pass by vineyards or other plantations, during the fertilization period. It's a small adjustment that makes all the difference.

I suggest bringing a cotton scarf to wrap around your neck in the morning or around your shoulders in the evening or, if necessary, to use to cover your head. I have one, a couple of meters long, which is very light and is also useful to keep flies away during the night in the hostel: I hang it above the bed (in hostels there are almost always bunk beds) and, by this, I create a protective screen, which lets air pass while keeping insects out.

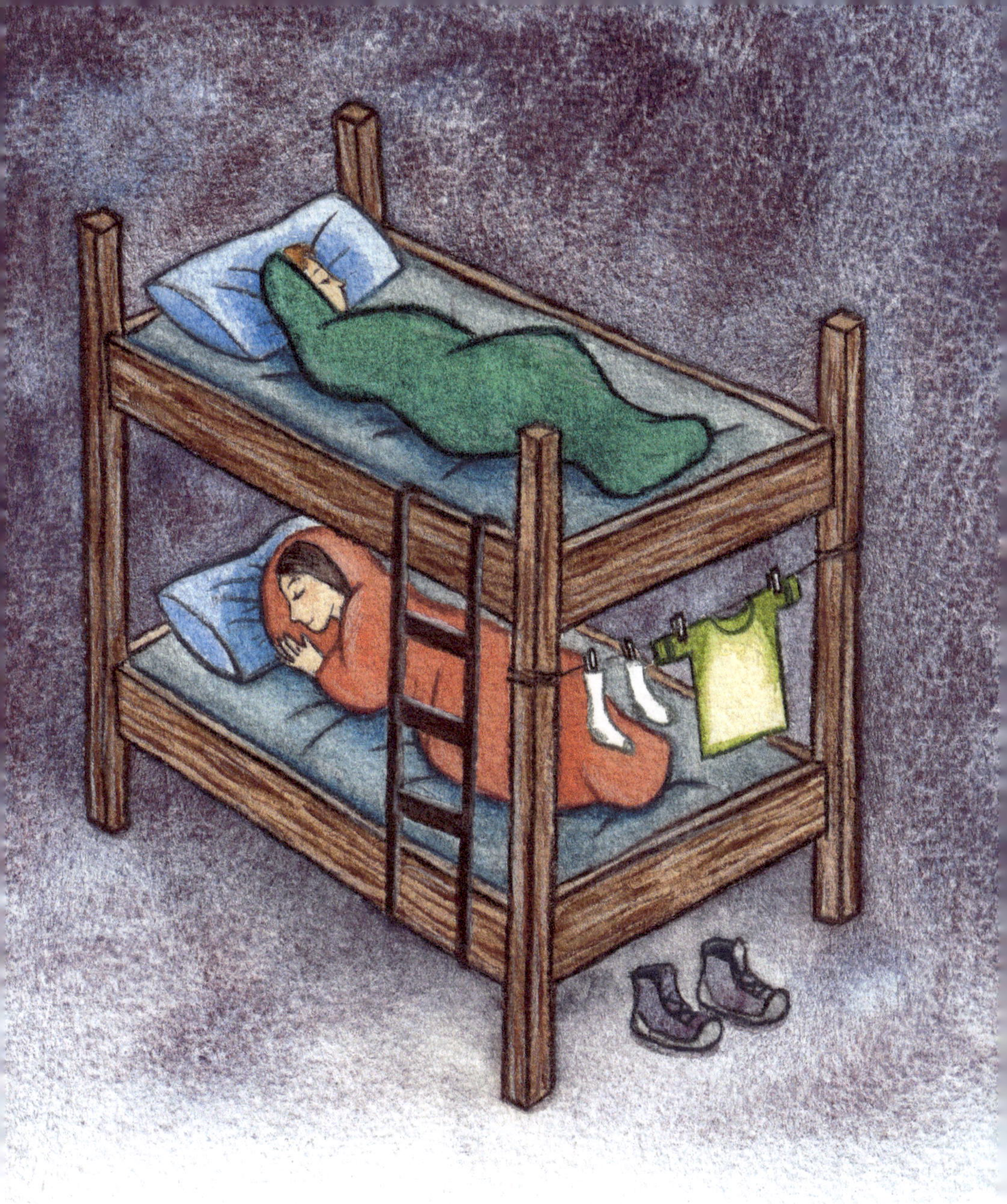

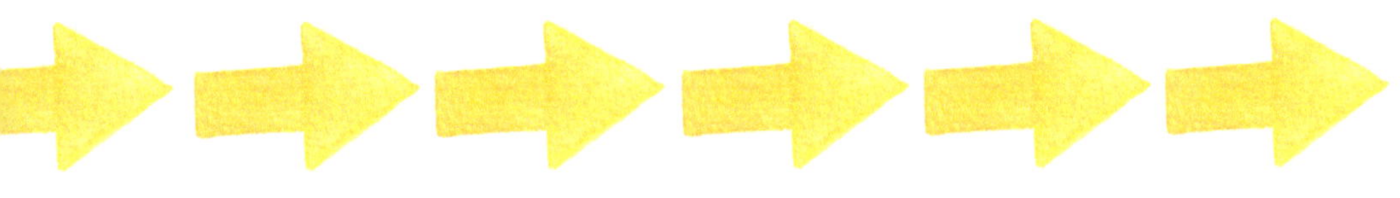

Before leaving for the Camino, you must obtain a credential: a piece of paper folded on itself into which you can enter your personal data (name, surname, nationality, identity document number and so on). The start date of the pilgrimage will be added and stamps will be added at each stage of the walk. They can be obtained from hostels and most of the bars and restaurants along the route. Each stamp will have a date and, once you arrive in Santiago, it will be possible to show proof of your journey at the office that issues the Compostela, a document attesting to the pilgrimage .

The credential is (unlike the Compostela) a mandatory document: without this piece of paper with stamps it is not possible to stay in public hostels dedicated to pilgrims. Naturally, it is possible to obtain stamps whether you are travelling on foot, on horseback or by bicycle. Nobody cares about how you are moving (you can also do the journey on a scooter), but it is important to know that to get the Compostela you need to cover at least the last hundred kilometres on foot, more if you use other means. Many pilgrims along the French Way decide to leave from Sarria, which makes that last stretch of the path very crowded. I recommend, as an alternative for those who want the Compostela at any cost, to take the English Way, which starts from Ferrol. It is a more peaceful and solitary journey compared to the last hundred kilometres of the French Way and the villages along the road are very characteristic. Once you arrive in Santiago by plane, you can take a bus to Ferrol, set off the next morning, and then leave by plane  from Santiago, once you have finished.

The credential is distributed by many churches in every country in Europe and you can apply directly online through their websites. Usually, a small offering is requested or in any case a small donation is very welcome if you go directly to the church to collect the credential. It is often possible to obtain a credential even at tourist offices, the main albergues and cathedrals. On the French Way, you will find it in Saint Jean Pied de Port (I picked up mine at the tourist office), in Burgos, in León and in Sarria. In Seville, I picked it up at the cathedral, before starting my walk along the Plata.

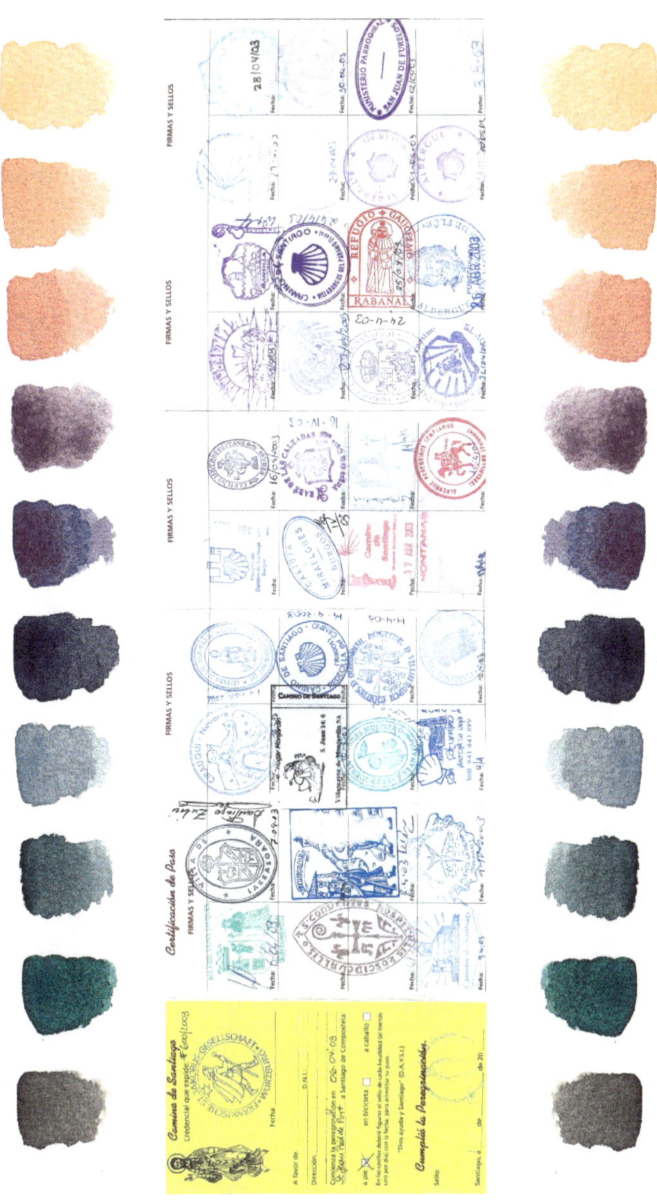

Of all the mistakes you can make when packing your backpack, overloading it is the most common. There isn't much time or energy to dedicate to reading works of fiction: reading tourist guides is completely normal, even books that talk about trekking. Carrying a Stephen King novel makes no sense. I met people who brought elegant clothes because "you never know", people who brought entire camping sets with them, including a stove and folding shower. During my first Camino, I made the mistake of carrying too many useless things.

This is an updated list of things I carry with me along my journeys, both in Spain and elsewhere. Clearly, if I decided to travel some stages in winter, I would dress according to the temperature and bring extra clothing with me, such as a hat, wool scarf and gloves. The list includes, for example, three shirts: two will go in the backpack and one will be worn. I suggest buying two t-shirts in technical fabric, to wear along the way, and one in cotton, to use for sleeping.

Clothing:

Three pairs of underwear
Three sports bras
Three t-shirts
Three pairs of socks (if using the double sock technique add a pair of thick socks)
A windbreaker with a fleece lining or a heavy sweatshirt
A pair of trousers with removable legs
Or a pair of leggings and two pairs of hiking shorts with pockets
A pair of flip flops
A pair of trekking sandals (if walking in summer)
A pair of hiking boots or a pair of trail running shoes
A hat with a peak or one with a wide brim
Sunglasses (and eyeglasses, if necessary)
A bandana
A light but long cotton scarf

Other necessary and/or useful items:

Technical backpack (I use a 25-litre backpack)
Foldable yoga mat
Sleeping bag
Travel bed sheet
Large water bottle
Technical shower towels: one small and one large
Technical waterproof bags
Trekking poles
Compass
Cell phone and charger
Swiss army knife
Strong rope and safety pins (for drying clothes)
Neutral bar soap
Toothpaste and toothbrush
Shampoo and shower gel
Total protection sun cream
Alcohol de romero (available in Spanish pharmacies)
Needle and thread
Gauze
Band-aids and disinfectant (disinfectant wipes are also very useful)
Mosquito and insect repellent spray
Flashlight
Identity card and health insurance
Lighter
Route guide with maps and tourist information
Diary
Pencil, pen, eraser and sharpener (optional: colours)

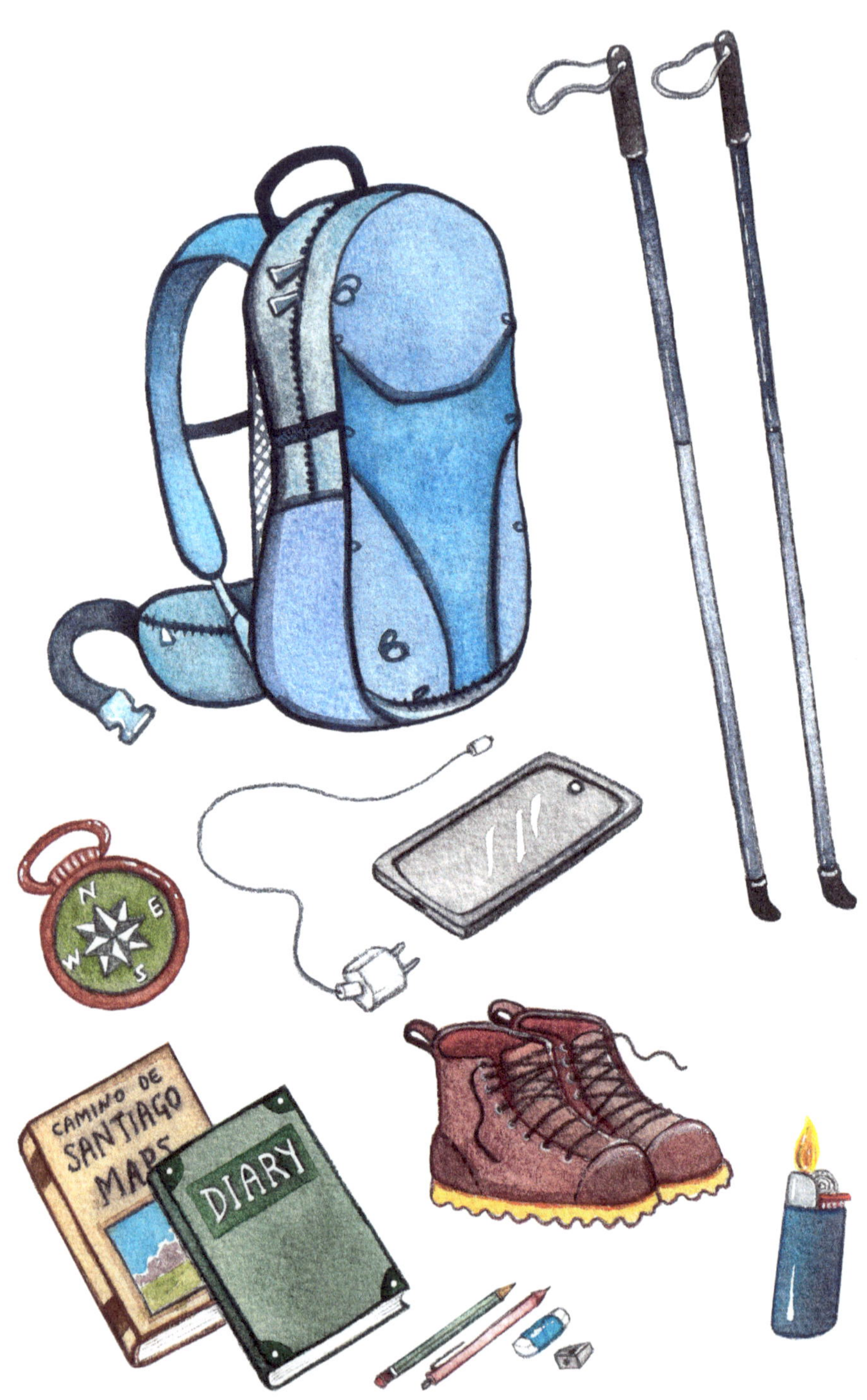
CAMINO DE
SANTIAGO
MAPS
DIARY
N
E
W
S

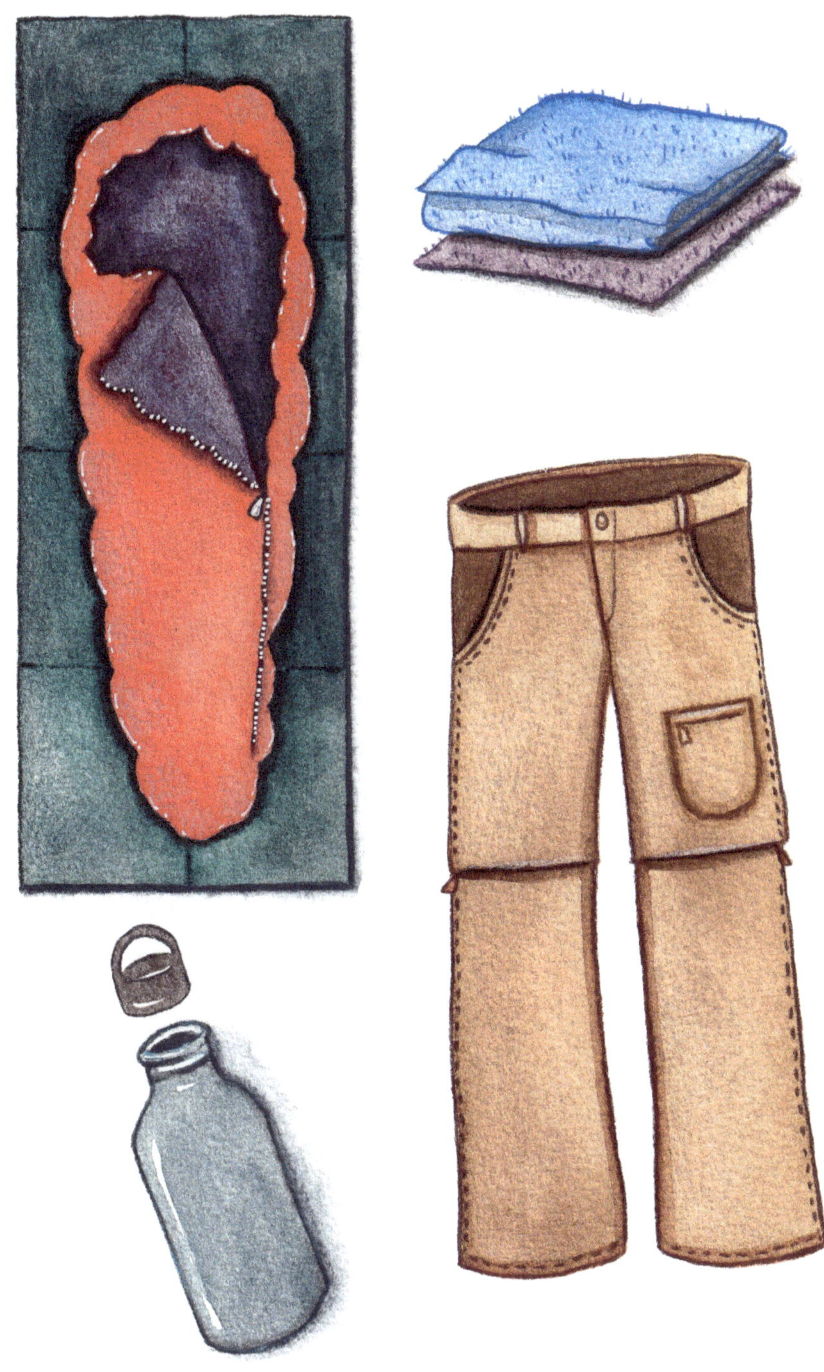

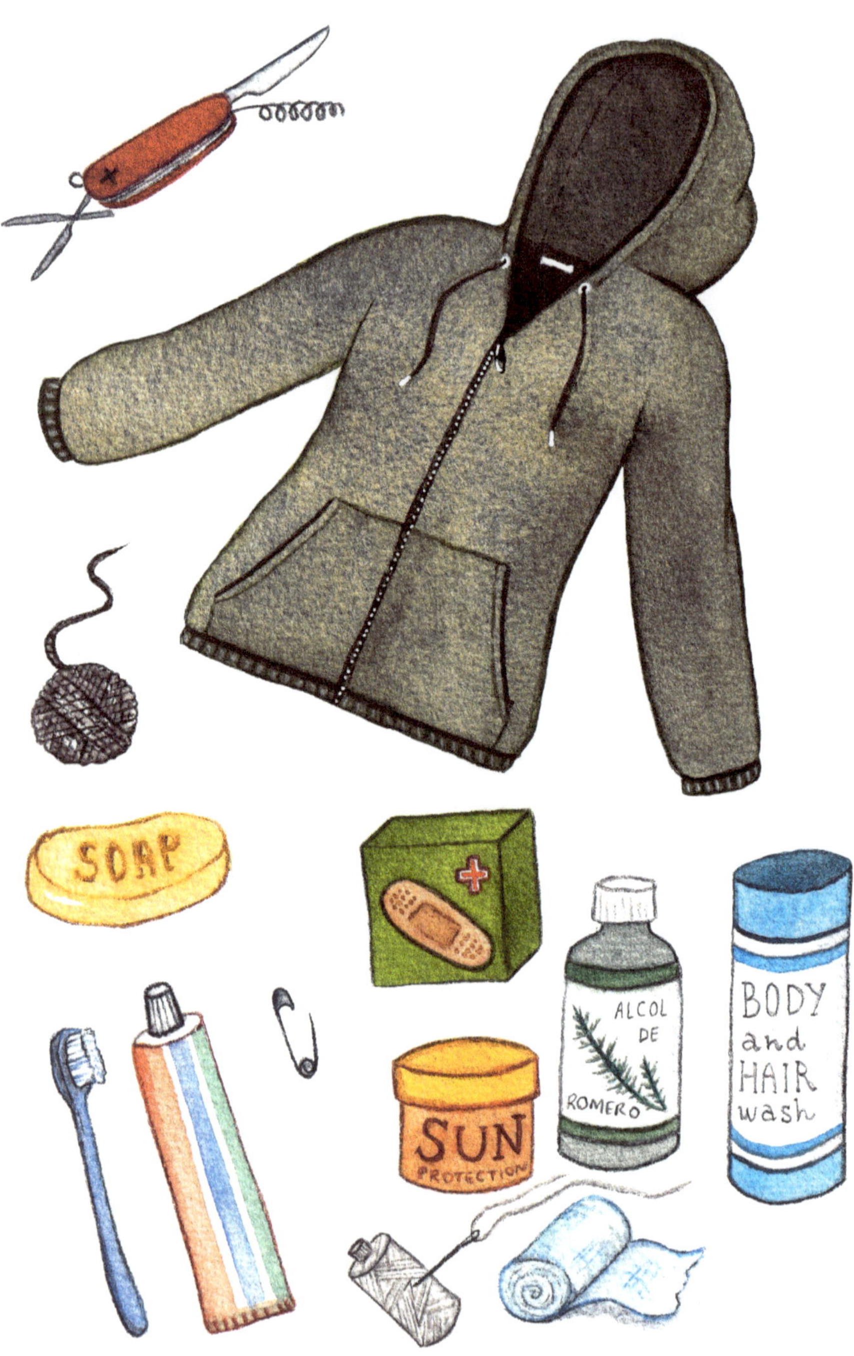
SORP
BODY
and
HAIR
wash
ALCOL
DE
ROMERO
SUN
PROTECTION

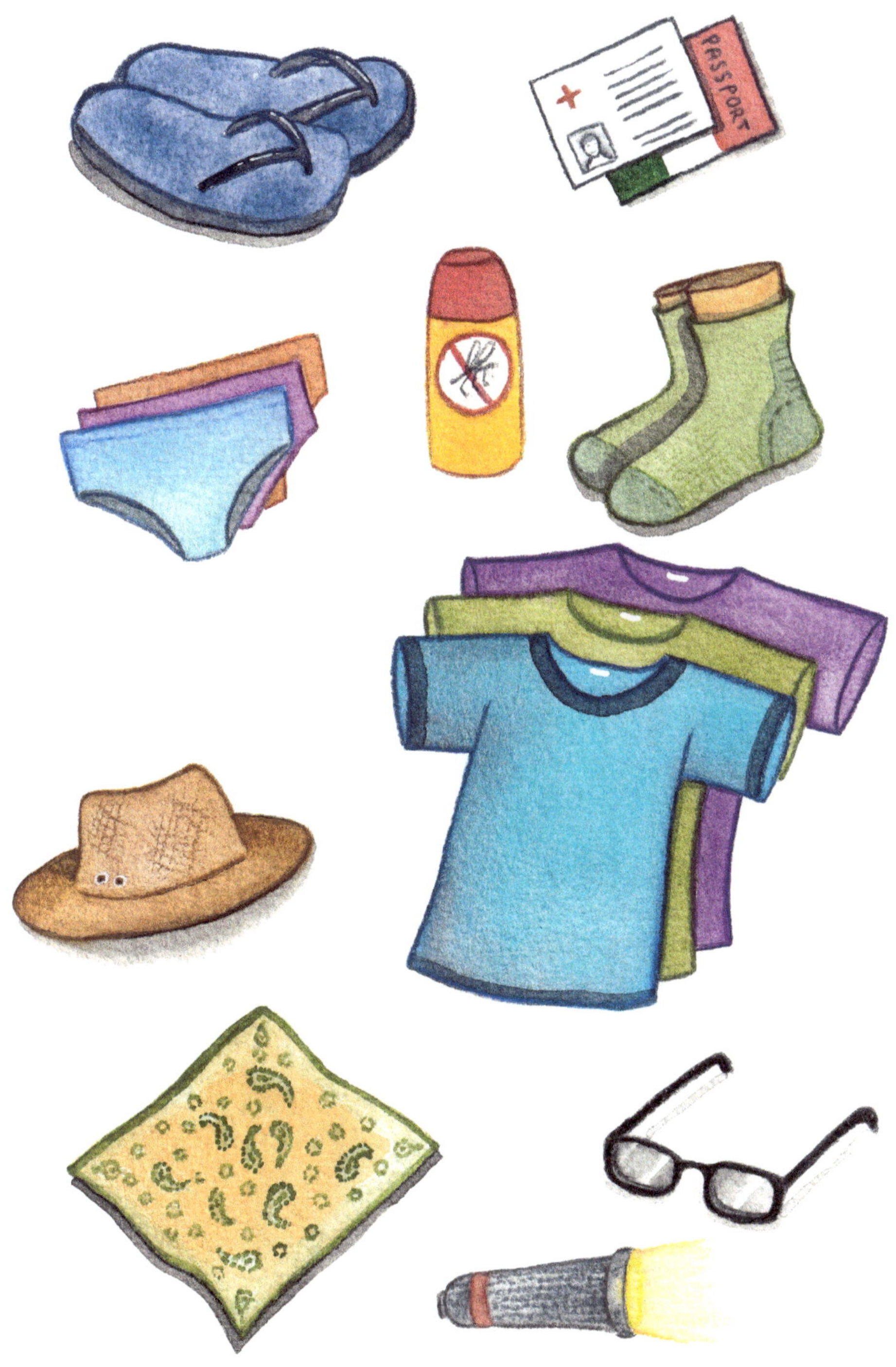

PASSPORT

One of the most important meals of the day is breakfast: especially when you have dozens of kilometres to travel ahead of you, it's a good habit to load up on energy. The Spanish breakfast is one of my all-time favourites. In addition to the classic croissant with coffee and milk (café con leche), you will almost always be offered orange juice (zumo de Naranja), toasted bread (tostadas) with tomato, olive oil, cheese and ham and the famous tortilla de patatas (a kind of tall potato omelette). In my experience, vegetarians might have some difficulty on the roads of Spain. It is rather rare to find vegetarian restaurants but it is almost always possible to order french fries or a portion of pimientos de Padrón (small fried green peppers). For vegans, it will be a challenge: my suggestion is to stock up on food in supermarkets. From personal experience, I recommend being very careful when ordering salad: although it is safe most of the time, it could happen in smaller villages or less attentive restaurants, to receive a dish in which the leaves have not been properly washed and the risk of gastroenteritis is quite high: I took a ride in an ambulance and spent a day in hospital near Ourense.

Absolutely worth trying: Iberian and Serrano ham (more delicate); Gazpacho (a cold, refreshing tomato soup), Paella, Fried calamari, Potatoes bravas, Pulpo a la Gallega, Chorizo, Fabada Asturiana, Catalan cream, Tarta de Santiago and much more that you will discover along the way. My advice is to be curious and, whenever it is possible, taste before deciding that a dish is not to your taste (I know that for some dishes it is impossible to do so – for example I don't like coriander, so I avoid dishes that contain it).

Usually, we need to stop somewhere for lunch: whether it's a supermarket offering the ingredients for lunch or whether it's a bar or a small restaurant, the best thing is sharing the moment with other pilgrims or with the locals. Especially the

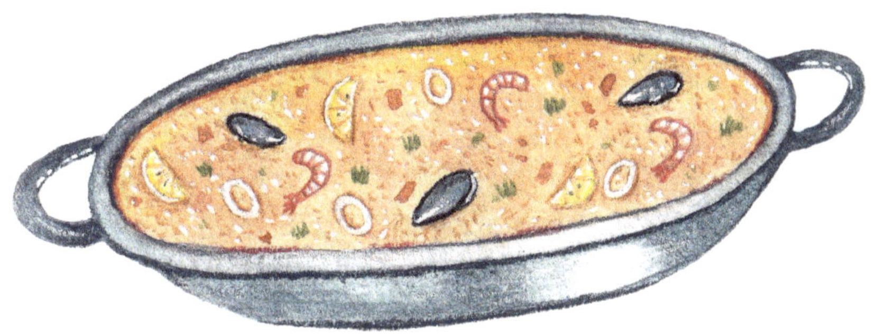

Paella

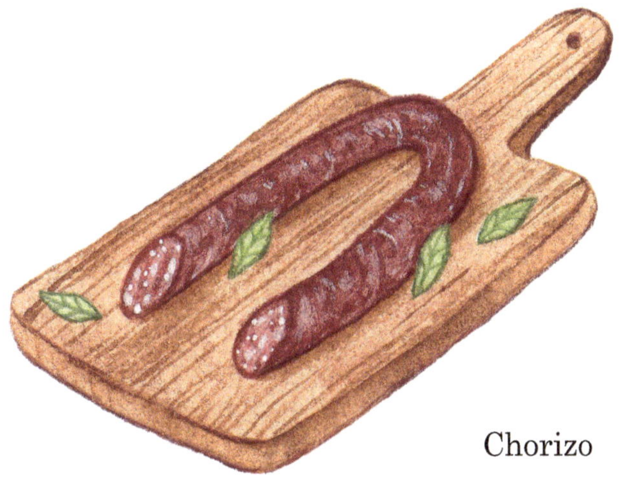

Chorizo

Tarta de Santiago

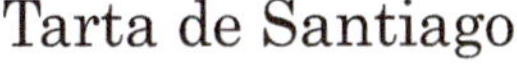

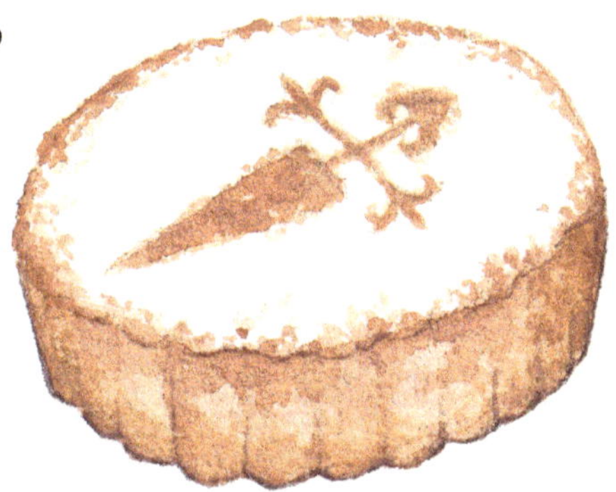

elderly are always welcoming and curious to know where you are coming from and how many kilometres you have travelled. Many locals are an inexhaustible source of information and the younger ones speak English without difficulty. My advice is not to eat too much in one meal but bring a couple of snacks with you: getting too heavy could lead to stomach problems down the road. Every two hours a small snack (for example toasted almonds or ice cream) helps keeping the energy and, above all, the morale high (most people argue when they're hungry).

For dinner, you will often find yourself sharing large tables with other pilgrims: if you decide to take advantage of some offers in the more organized albergues, know that you will often find yourself eating the same dishes, simple and cheap. The cost is low but so is the variety. However, I don't think it will be an insurmountable inconvenience, given that after many kilometres on foot you will have an intense hunger that will make you appreciate even the simplest dish of pasta with sauce.

A great way to make friends along the way is to cook for your travel companions. Depending on the type of hostel where you decide to stay, it is possible that there is a nicely equipped kitchen, sometimes with some basic ingredients (such as dry spices, salt, oil and vinegar) left by the hospitalero or by some pilgrim who passed through on one of the previous days. If you find yourself in a situation where you can prepare a nice spaghetti dinner for everyone, do it without hesitation! In local supermarkets it is easy to find basic products, such as potatoes, onions, ready-made sauces and cheese. Don't be afraid to spend a few extra Euros to feed your traveling companions: it will be a moment of community that will stay in your heart.

Be careful with alcohol consumption: drinking too much while walking could lead to various types of inconveniences, both for you and for those travelling alongside you. Exercise moderation or, better yet, avoid drinking alcohol altogether. For some people the Camino is a perfect time to say goodbye to alcohol and make room for a healthier lifestyle. Look around and make sure you don't offer wine to people who are trying to break free from an alcohol addiction: along the roads leading to Santiago you will find many people who have embarked on a journey towards sobriety and it would be very rude and inappropriate to make them drink.

Remember that, once you arrive in Obradoiro square, in front of the cathedral of Santiago, it is strictly forbidden to uncork bottles and toast the success of the undertaking (it is also forbidden to eat or drink in general). The city of Santiago is full of restaurants, pubs and bars where you can party: respect the historic site of the cathedral, whether you are a believer or not.

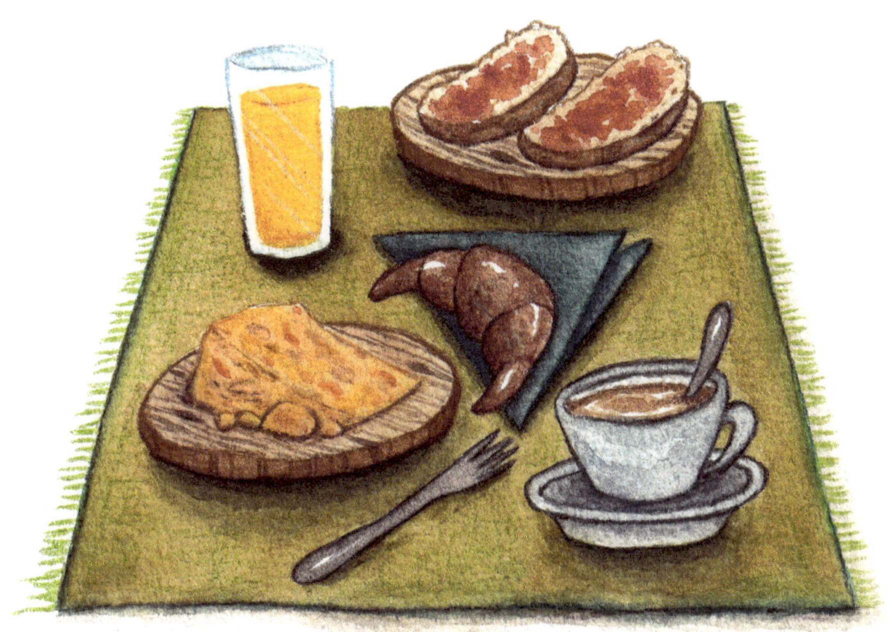

For those who want to have the most authentic experience, albergues are the best places to stay overnight. They are houses often managed by the municipality or the local parish, open to all pilgrims and equipped with numerous beds. In most cases a donation is expected: an offering that covers the costs of cleaning and management of the premises. The style in which these places are furnished can vary greatly and the same goes for the type of hospitality. On my numerous journeys, I have stayed overnight in a former schoolhouse where there were only gym mats to sleep on, sheds in the middle of the countryside with folding beds like military cots and "luxury" hostels where even cloth sheets and clean towels, as well as wonderful breakfasts, were welcoming me. Every day you spend on the path, you will have to make choices: sometimes the albergue might not be adequate for you and you will reluctantly decide to walk another five kilometres in the hope of finding a better one. On other days, you will be spoiled with options (especially in larger cities, such as Burgos or León).

The French Way of St. James is the most popular and, consequently, the economy of the villages that this route passes through is focussed primarily on welcoming pilgrims. Be careful not to be taken for a ride by crafty hospitaleros who ask you astronomical sums without offering you the services you need: always ask if there are sheets on the beds, if there is hot water for the shower, or if it is possible to have a single room. More often than not it is and I can guarantee you that it will be a blessing to be able to sometimes sleep without a snoring neighbour or the smell of someone who doesn't wash. There are those who walk the Camino and always stay at a hotel. If you already know that you can afford it and you want to have more privacy, don't hesitate: your bed in the hostel will be given to someone else and everyone will be happy.

If you are a pilgrim by bike, make sure not to occupy the last bed in a small village hostel: for you, travelling ten kilometres more is not the end of the world, for those who walk it's a whole different story (I speak from experience, having covered parts of the journey by bicycle).

Showing education and respect is fundamental:
• Don't leave garbage everywhere
• Clean your cutlery and plates in the albergues.
• Shower and wash your clothes daily (yes, every day!).
• Don't be noisy when other pilgrims go to sleep and try to be quiet in the morning if you get up before the others.
• If you have the opportunity to help a pilgrim who is suffering, try to lend a hand (offer some plasters, tissues or an aspirin).

Receiving care from a stranger is one of the most intense moments of the entire pilgrimage experience and makes us, for a moment, see the world with a more serene vision. Once you arrive in Santiago, remember that you can also continue walking! You can, for example, go to Finisterre or La Coruña, which can be reached in a few days' walk.

Once you get home, go to the bookshop and look for other routes: Europe is full of more or less well-known routes, which connect us to wonderful cities passing through breath-taking landscapes.

Buen Camino!

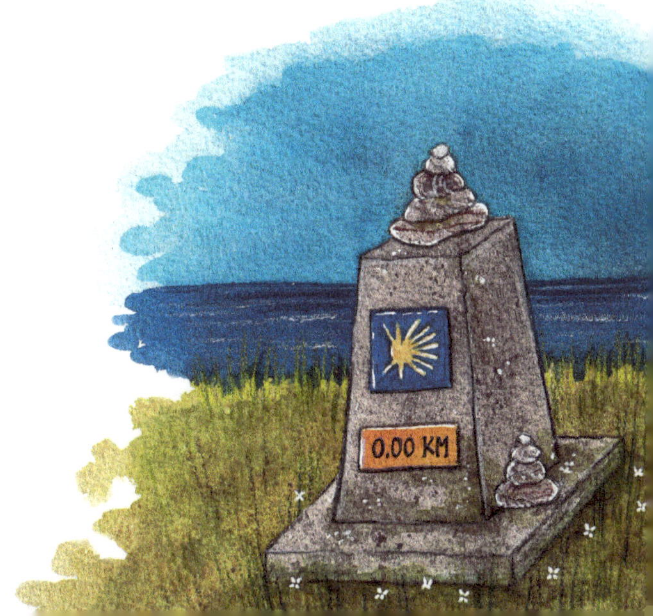